British Medical Association
Board of Science

# Over-the-counter medication

May 2005

# Editorial board

British Library Cataloguing-in-Publication Data.
A catalogue record for this book is available from the British Library.

ISBN: 0-9548965-2-1
Cover photograph: Getty Images Creative
Printed by the BMA publications unit

# Board of Science

This report was prepared under the auspices of the Board of Science of the British Medical Association, whose membership for 2004/2005 was as follows:

Approval for publication as a BMA policy report was recommended by BMA Board of Professional Activities on 6 May 2005.

For further information about the editorial secretariat or Board members please contact the science and education department: info.science@bma.org.uk

# Acknowledgements

The association is very grateful for the help provided by the BMA committees and many outside experts and organisations. We would particularly like to thank:

- Professor Colin Bradley, Professor of General Practice, University College, Cork, Southern Ireland

- Professor Tony Avery, Professor of Primary Health Care, School of Community Health Sciences, Division of Primary Care, Nottingham University Medical School

- Dr Ross Taylor, retired Senior Lecturer (Clinical Consultant) Dept of General Practice and Primary Care, University of Aberdeen

- Helen Tyrrell, Director of Voluntary Health Scotland

## About the authors

Alison Blenkinsopp is Professor of the Practice of Pharmacy at Keele University's Department of Medicines Management. She has researched and written widely about self-care and OTC medication. She is lead author of *Symptoms in the pharmacy: a guide to the management of common illness,* a standard academic text for pharmacists now in its fifth edition and translated into several languages. She was a member of the Committee on Safety of Medicines from 1999-2005, where she had a particular interest in the reclassification of medicines. She remains a member of the BNF Committee, to which she was appointed in 1989.

Christine Bond is Professor of Primary Care (Pharmacy), and Deputy Head of Department, in the Department of General Practice and Primary Care, University of Aberdeen. She is also a Consultant in Pharmaceutical Public Health, with NHS Grampian and Editor of the International Journal of Pharmacy Practice. Her research concerns the optimum use of both prescribed and OTC medicines and the contribution of community pharmacy to the primary healthcare agenda. She has published widely in this area. She is a member of the Scottish Executive of the RPSGB, the Main Research Ethics Committee for Scotland, the Health Services Research Committee of the Chief Scientist Office, Scottish Executive Health Department, and the National Pharmaceutical Forum (Scotland).

# Foreword

The Board of Science, a standing committee of the British Medical Association (BMA) provides an interface between the medical profession, the government and the public. One major aim of the board is to contribute to the improvement of public health, and it has developed a wide range of policies on the health of specific groups such as children and the elderly.

At the BMA's 2004 annual representative meeting a motion on over-the-counter (OTC) medication was debated and referred to the Board of Science for further consideration. In commissioning this report, the Board decided that given the many changes in the field of OTC medication, a report setting the specific issues within the wider context would be valuable.

Increasing patient involvement in the diagnosis and treatment of common ailments has led to a greater interest in and encouragement of self-care and an increase in the use of non-prescription drug products commonly referred to as OTC medications. OTC medications now account for about £2 billion of the £11 billion spent in the UK on medication and may be used to prevent, treat or cure ailments from cardiovascular conditions (eg simvastatin) to common aches and pains (eg paracetamol). The largest expenditures are for analgesics and skin treatments.[1]

The availability of OTC medications has increased both through the creation of new preparations and the reclassification of existing substances. Between 1983 and 1999 there were 72 reclassifications from POM to P (Royal Pharmaceutical Society of Great Britain 2000). The government has recently pledged to double the rate of reclassification and work to increase the availability of OTCs for common complaints.[2]

The purpose of this report is to provide an analysis of the current trends in OTC medications, as well as current treatment and prevention strategies using OTC medications, followed by recommendations for improving these strategies. This information will be of use to a variety of groups including health professionals seeking advice on helping patients and policymakers seeking to improve or introduce legislation in this area.

---

[1] PAGB. OTC Medicines Sales figures 2004. www.pagb.org.uk (Accessed 23 May 2005)

[2] PAGB. OTC Medicines Sales figures 2003.
www.pagb.org.uk/media/downloads/downloads.asp?mode=doc&id=223 (Accessed 18 August 2004)

# Contents

**1. The scope of OTC medication**

1.1 Legal classification of OTC medicines

1.2 Use of OTC medication

1.3 The evidence base for OTC medicines

1.4 Switching of medicines from prescription to OTC

1.5 Government policy on OTC medication

1.6 Doctors' attitudes to OTC medication

1.7 Access to OTC medicines

**2. Patient/user perspectives**

2.1 Decision making about OTC medicines

2.2 Influences on OTC use

2.3 Older people and OTC medicines

2.4 Children and OTC medicines

2.5 Compliance with OTC medicines

**3. Balance of benefits and risks**

3.1 Risk of adverse events

3.2 Impact of OTC medication on diagnosis

3.3 Misuse

3.4 Further investigation required

3.5 Parenteral use

3.6 Availability versus control

**4. Role of professionals**

4.1 Pharmacists and their staff

4.2 General practitioners

4.3 Nurses

4.4 Collaborative care

**5. Information and communication**

5.1 Pharmacoepidemiology of OTC medication use

5.2 Information for the public

5.3 Records of OTC purchases

5.4 Shared patient records

**6. Conclusions**

**7. Recommendations**

**Glossary**

**References**

**Sources of further information**

# Introduction

Over-the-counter (OTC) medicines have traditionally been used to treat self-limiting minor ailments. The scope for treating such conditions has been extended by the switch from prescription to OTC status of effective treatments and this is likely to continue. The global trend towards, and encouragement of, increased self-care including self-management of long-term conditions, is likely to affect the range and availability of OTC medication in the future. A strategic approach will be needed to integrate OTC medication with the wider NHS.

Like all treatment interventions, OTC medicines bring both benefits and risks. Potential benefits to the public include enabling people to take control of their own illnesses and rapid and convenient access to treatments. Potential risks include adverse effects and the possible misuse of certain medicines. Potential benefits to the healthcare system include more efficient use of physician capacity through the transfer of consultations about minor ailments to pharmacists and nurses, as well as increased individual responsibility and empowerment in the context of minor ailments. Shaw and Baker have suggested the term 'Involved Patients' to denote active involvement in treatment choices and self-management of health (Shaw & Baker 2004) and this is apposite for self-medication with OTC medicines.

Health professionals need to routinely ask about any OTC medicines the patient has tried or is taking. If more OTC medicines intended for long-term or intermittent use are to become available, safety would be improved by documenting the use of such medicines. Until shared electronic access to information becomes possible, a patient-held record would be a means whereby different people involved in the patient's care could see information about OTC use. Challenges inherent in such a record are its acceptability to the public, as well as the documentation of third party purchases, or those purchases that are to stock the home medicine chest. Appropriate information provided on medicine packaging and patient information leaflets should be used to improve the public understanding of the benefits and risks of OTC medicines. User testing of both is essential to ensure this objective is met.

# 1. The scope of OTC medication

## 1.1 Legal classification of medicines

The UK has three legal categories of medicines:

| | | | |
|---|---|---|---|
| Prescription only medicine | POM | Requires a prescription from specified health professional/s | 'In the dispensary' |
| Pharmacy medicines | P | Must be sold by, or under the supervision of, a registered pharmacist | 'Behind-the-counter' |
| General sales list medicine | GSL | Available from any sales outlet, eg garage, newsagent | 'Off-the-shelf' |

The P category requires supervision by a pharmacist, and might be thought of as the 'behind-the-counter' category to differentiate it from 'off-the-shelf' medicines (Fenichel 2004). The OTC market includes the P and GSL categories, and also herbal and homeopathic medicines, which are currently not regulated under the same system. In the UK, medicines in the P category can only be sold 'under the supervision' of a pharmacist, from registered pharmacy premises, whereas the GSL products can be sold both from pharmacies, without the supervision requirement, and from any retail outlet. The pharmacy supervision requirement has been interpreted in its strictest sense with a requirement for the pharmacist to be both present in the pharmacy and aware of all such sales. To some extent this has limited the pharmacist taking on other duties and thus has led to a review of alternative arrangements as part of a wider consultation on making the best use of the pharmacy workforce (Department of Health 2004). One option suggested is that the law should be amended so that the supply of P or prescribed POM medicines no longer requires the pharmacist's presence in the pharmacy at all times. At the time of writing the outcome of the consultation is not known.

## 1.2 Use of OTC medication

Self-care occurs in over 80 per cent of episodes of common ailments (BMRB 1997 Everyday Health Care – A consumer study of self-medication in Great Britain). Table 1 shows the ailments that this study found were most frequently experienced by adults.

Clearly there are some seasonal changes in the pattern of episodes of illness, but this study provides a useful snapshot. It is important to note that the methodology captured all ailments experienced, not only those where the respondent self-treated. In just over half the cases where adults experienced an ailment no treatment was used. Where treatment was used (46 per cent of episodes), it was a prescription medicine already available in the house in around a quarter of cases, an OTC medicine in over half, and a 'home remedy' (for example a hot water bottle) in the remainder of episodes.

**Table 1: Ailments most commonly experienced in the previous two weeks (adults)**

| Ailment | Percentage of people reporting self-treatment |
|---|---|
| 1. Tiredness | 40% |
| 2. Headache | 33% |
| 3. Muscular aches/pains | 29% |
| 3. Sleeping problems | 23% |
| 4. Stiffness in joints | 22% |
| 5. Back problems | 20% |
| 6. Bruises | 17% |
| 7. Stress/anxiety | 17% |
| 8. Feeling low/depressed | 16% |
| 9. Indigestion/heartburn | 16% |
| 10. Minor cuts/grazes | 16% |

**Source: BRMB, Everyday Health Care 1997**

The ailments that people in the UK say they are most likely to self-treat are shown in table 2. These ailments are a subset of those that are experienced and there are therefore differences between the ailments listed in table 1 and those in table 2. Three of the 10 ailments most likely to be self-treated, for example, were painful conditions (headache, migraine, period pain). Clearly the availability of more OTC treatments has the potential to increase the range of symptoms being self-treated. The switch of medicines from POM to P is a key development in this respect.

**Table 2: Ailments for which people in the UK report treating themselves rather than seeking a consultation with a doctor (n = 2,000)**

| Ailment | Percentage of people reporting self-treatment |
|---|---|
| 1. Headache | 80% |
| 2. Athlete's foot | 79% |
| 3. Dandruff | 73% |
| 4. Heartburn | 62% |
| 5. Migraine | 62% |
| 6. Period pain | 61% |
| 7. Colds | 60% |
| 8. Coughs | 56% |
| 9. Mouth ulcers | 51% |
| 10. Acid stomach | 50% |

Source: PRISM (Progressive Research In Self-Medication) 94. London: Readers Digest, 1994

While sleeping problems, stress/anxiety and feeling low/depressed featured in the list of ailments most commonly experienced, they did not appear in the list of ailments for self-treatment. This may, to some extent, reflect methodological differences between the two studies but is also likely to be because most treatments for these problems are POM.

Studies from other countries are potentially useful points of comparison, although the effects of cultural differences and different healthcare systems must be remembered. However, in general, such population-based surveys show substantial levels of OTC use. A German survey, for example, found that 29.9 per cent of men and 41.2 per cent of women had used an OTC medicine in the previous week (Beitz et al 2004). This usage was additional to prescribed medicines in 12.3 per cent and 29.3 per cent respectively. Vitamins, minerals and analgesics were the most frequently reported products used and the most commonly reported indication was 'prevention'.

Findings from studies of patients seeing a doctor or nurse in primary care indicate that considerable numbers of people are taking both prescribed and OTC medicines. One UK survey of 2,765 patients presenting for consultations at six medical practices asked about regular medicine use and found that in the UK 55.1 per cent took regular prescribed medication and 24.6 per cent used OTC medicines regularly (Bradley et al 1998). In a US study of consultations in primary care 57 per cent of patients reported using one or more OTC medications during the previous month (Sleath et al). Although this percentage seems high it is likely to reflect regular, occasional and acute use of OTCs.

## 1.3 The evidence base for OTC medicines

Some health professionals question whether OTC medicines are effective. The picture is complex and at present the evidence base is not readily accessible. There is also the argument that treatment is about more than the evidence base; as a GP responding to the findings of a systematic review put it, *'Evidence based medicine has much to offer but please don't let us confuse pharmacological efficacy with the real world of managing human emotions alongside physical illness'* (Checkland 2002).

Nevertheless, health professionals recommending OTC medicines need to be able to easily access and consider the available evidence. For newer OTC medicines, including those switched from POM to P, the regulatory system requires evidence of safety and efficacy; this is generally provided by the pharmaceutical industry and much of the available evidence is likely to have come from the use of the medicine as a POM. Independently conducted systematic reviews of evidence are also available for some such medicines, for example, on the effectiveness of orally and intra-vaginally administered imidazoles and triazoles in the treatment of vaginal thrush (Watson et al 2001).

For some older medicines there are few or no clinical trials to provide evidence and it is unlikely that such studies will now be conducted. Perhaps the most controversial treatments in this respect are those for upper respiratory tract infections. Consumers continue to purchase products to treat coughs and colds despite little formal evidence of effectiveness in either adults (Schroeder et al 2002) or children (Hay et al 2004) in the outcomes measured in clinical trials (for example, duration of symptoms). These may not necessarily be the same outcomes that medicines users themselves might select (for example, a small amount of relief from troublesome symptoms) but no published research has explored this. With the exception of a small number of simple medicines, the majority of treatments for coughs and colds are blacklisted and not available on the NHS for this reason.

Systematic reviews have also shown that the doses of adjuvant drugs, eg codeine in OTC combination analgesic are too low to provide an analgesics effect yet they continue to be widely advertised and used by the public (Li Wan Po et al 1996). This may lead to individuals exceeding the OTC dose in order to match the dose of a product previously obtained on prescription, or to achieve the required analgesia. There is however no published research to confirm or refute this.

Those health professionals and consumers who are sufficiently determined and skilled in accessing information can draw together research findings from multiple primary and secondary sources (for example Cochrane Collaboration, Best Treatments, NeLH, PRODIGY, NICE) to put together the pieces of the evidence jigsaw. Bringing together existing evidence on OTC medicines could support decision making by both healthcare providers and the public. Methods to support decision making in clinical practice are discussed later (see Role of professionals).

## 1.4 Switching of medicines from prescription to OTC

Medicines may be switched from POM to P and from P to GSL status. There is a general recognition that when any new medicine first receives a licence there is a need for POM control so that experience of use and safety in large numbers of patients can be gained under medical supervision. However, many POM medicines might later be suitable for OTC availability. There is a worldwide trend in switching medicines from POM to P and the European view is that 'no medicine should remain POM unless necessary for reasons of safety'. Key medicines switched from POM to P since 1983 in the UK are shown in table 3.

**Table 3 – Key UK POM to P switches 1983-2005**

| 1983 | Ibuprofen<br>Loperamide<br>Terfenadine |
|------|-----------------------------------------|
| 1987 | Topical hydrocortisone for dermatitis |
| 1991 | Nicotine replacement therapy (NRT) |
| 1992 | Clotrimazole for vaginal thrush |
| 1993 | Topical aciclovir for cold sores<br>Cetirizine; loratadine |
| 1994 | Cimetidine; famotidine<br>Beclometasone nasal spray<br>Topical hydrocortisone for eczema<br>Steroid-containing suppositories for haemorrhoids |
| 1995 | Fluconazole for vaginal thrush |
| 1998 | Mebeverine for Irritable Bowel Syndrome |
| 2001 | Levonorgestrel emergency hormonal contraception |
| 2002 | Fluticasone nasal spray |
| 2003 | Omeprazole |
| 2004 | Simvastatin |
| 2005 | Chloramphenicol eye drops |

Source: PAGB Self Care Review 2004

The EC guidance for retaining the POM status of a medicine is explicit and enshrined in a European Directive (European Community 1992), later revised (European Parliament and Council 2001). This declared that no medicine should remain a POM unless:

- there is direct or indirect danger to health if the medicine is used without medical supervision (for example the adverse drug reaction (ADR) profile needs a doctor to assess risk–benefit, or misdiagnosis might lead to the patient being put at risk)
- the medicine is frequently used incorrectly leading to direct or indirect danger to health (eg products liable to misuse)
- the activity of the drug or the side effects require further investigation
- the drug is parenterally administered.

An application is made with supporting data on safety and efficacy. It is then considered by the UK regulator (the Medicines and Healthcare products Regulatory Agency (MHRA), formerly the Medicines Control Agency (MCA) through its Committee on Safety of Medicines, which advises ministers. Aronson recently suggested that 'essential' criteria for a switch should be the diagnosis, efficacy and safety, with improved accessibility, rapid accessibility and shifting costs as 'desirable' criteria (Aronson 2004).

Despite common principles for switching medicines from POM to P the availability of medicines varies considerably between countries (table 4).

**Table 4: OTC availability in selected countries**

|  | Australia | Belgium | New Zealand | Portugal | Singapore | UK | USA |
|---|---|---|---|---|---|---|---|
| Chloramphenical (topical, eye) | POM | OTC | POM | OTC | POM | OTC | POM |
| Codeine | OTC | OTC | OTC | POM | OTC | OTC | POM |
| Fluconazole (oral) | OTC | POM | OTC | POM | POM | OTC | POM |
| Levonorgestrel | OTC | OTC | OTC | POM | POM | OTC | POM |
| Naproxen | OTC | OTC | OTC | OTC | OTC | POM | OTC |
| Omeprazole | POM | POM | POM | POM | POM | OTC | OTC |
| Orlistat | OTC | POM | OTC | POM | POM | POM | POM |
| Salbutamol | OTC | POM | OTC | POM | OTC | POM | POM |
| Simvastatin | POM | POM | POM | POM | POM | OTC | POM |

In some countries, for example the USA, there is only the basic division between those medicines that can be obtained on prescription and those that can be purchased in any retail outlet. Non-steroidal anti-inflammatory drugs (NSAID) are an interesting example. In the UK, ibuprofen is the only oral NSAID that can be purchased OTC, and in non-pharmacy outlets the pack size is limited to 16 doses. UK visitors to the USA are therefore surprised to see a range of oral non-steroidal anti-inflammatories (ketoprofen, naproxen, as well as ibuprofen) on supermarket shelves, in products for adults and children, and in pack sizes of up to several hundred tablets. Australia and New Zealand, in contrast, have four legal categories including a sub-category of pharmacist-only medicines where the pharmacist's personal involvement is required in each sale (for example, newly-deregulated medicines such as orlistat). There are also variations between European countries. In Italy, for example, there are prescription only medicines, SOP (senza obbligo di prescrizione), and a category called PDB (prodotto da banco) commonly known as OTC. Both the SOP and PDB medicines, however, are only available through pharmacies and sold by the pharmacist; the difference is that the OTC medicines can be advertised directly to the public, and displayed in areas for customer self-selection, if the pharmacist so wishes. A similar position exists in France and some other European countries. In the Netherlands however, there are only POM and OTC. Pharmacies focus on POM medicines, and have a minority role in the sale of OTCs, 75 per cent of which are sold from 'drogisten' (chemists) which also sell a wide range of products including toothpaste, and body care products. The Netherlands abolished its equivalent of the pharmacy only category and there are now moves to reinstate it to enable a new 'breed' of OTC medicines to be deregulated from prescription controls and used for self-treatment of long-term conditions.

An important implication of these differences is that deregulation from POM may be judged inappropriate in countries where there is no P category or equivalent. A recent example was the FDA's decision against OTC status for lovastatin because of concerns that consumers could not safely self-assess whether the treatment would be appropriate and safe for them.

It is unlikely that there will be total agreement across Europe in drug classification in the near future, although recent changes may lead to greater congruity. There are now procedures for mutual recognition, which 'enables manufacturers to seek simultaneous marketing authorisation in two or more member states known as the Concerned Member States (CMS) providing they have an existing marketing authorisation for that drug in at least one member state, known as the reference member state (RMS)' (Abraham and Lewis 1999). Some of the differences of individual classification may also be historical. It is possible that some currently available GSL medicines would not have that status if they were assessed against today's criteria, for example, aspirin may be associated with severe adverse events such as gastro-intestinal bleeding, or misuse/overuse as in the analgesic dependent headache.

The UK is currently the world leader in increasing the range and availability of OTC medicines. The regulators, working with professional bodies (pharmacy, medicine and nursing) and lay representatives, produced a list of medicines that might potentially be switched from POM to P (RPSGB 2001a) together with a strategic framework to support such switches eg protocols to identify people eligible for treatment, and training for pharmacists and their staff (RPSGB 2001b). The list of potential switches was wide ranging and included medicines for several long-term conditions such as hypertension and asthma.

POM to P switching introduces new treatment options for the public (for example, a medicine for a condition not previously treatable with OTCs) and sometimes new treatment indications for existing OTCs. The switching of medicines from P to GSL generally receives less attention but is an important component of UK policy on improving access to medicines. GSL status acknowledges that there are times when pharmacies are not open but people still need to be able to access OTC medicines. This is particularly an issue outside of usual business hours (typically between 6pm and 9am, and on Sundays). The criterion for switching from P to GSL is that the medicine 'can with reasonable safety be sold or supplied otherwise than by or under the supervision of a pharmacist' (Medicines Act 1968, section 51).

Experience of use as a POM medicine contributes to decisions regarding deregulating medicines to P status, and in turn experience of use as a P medicine informs decisions about total deregulation to GSL status. The regulator states that, 'Pharmacy medicines which have been safely used for several years may be suitable for general sale and may be reclassified as GSL' (MHRA 2005). However, there is currently no systematic collection of data on the appropriateness and safety of P medicine usage, and such evidence is largely anecdotal.

## 1.5 Government policy on OTC medication

In the blueprint for NHS modernisation the NHS Plan included a target relating to the public being able to 'get the right medicine at the right time' (NHS Plan 2000). This theme related to both prescribed and OTC medicines. In relation to OTC medicines there was a target of 10 switches (including both POM to P and P to GSL) each year. Table 5 shows the number of switches made since the introduction by the MHRA in 2002 of the new process for dealing with switch applications.

**Table 5: Applications to reclassify a medicine (ARM) consultations by the MHRA 2002-2004**

| Year | POM to P | P to GSL |
|------|----------|----------|
| 2002 | Fluticasone nasal spray | Ketoconazole 2% shampoo |
| | Vivioptal capsules (multivitamin/multimineral) | Minoxidil 2% lotion |
| | | Pharmaton capsules (ginseng/multivitamin/multimineral) |
| | | Topical hydrocortisone 1% (for bites and stings) |
| | | Beclometasone nasal spray (adults, hayfever) |
| 2003 | Omeprazole 10mg | NiQuitin 4mg lozenge (2 products) (nicotine) |
| | Topical diclofenac (new indication – non-serious arthritic pain) | Hyoscine butylbromide |
| | Diclofenac spraygel | Dioralyte Relief (2 products) |
| | Scopoderm patch (1.5mg hyoscine) | Clotrimazole cream + pessary |
| | Zocor Heart Pro (simvastatin 10mg) | Cetirizine tablets; cetirizine syrup |
| | | Nurofen Cold & Flu (200mg ibuprofen + pseudoephedrine 30mg)* |
| | | Anbesol (lidocaine; chlorocresol; cetylpyridinium) |
| | | Terbinafine cream; terbinafine spray |
| 2004 | Chloramphenical eye drops | Aciclovir cream 5% |
| | | Wasp-eze (benzocaine 1%; mepyramine maleate 0.5%) |
| | | Topical diclofenac 1.16% |
| | | Germoloids HC spray (hydrocortisone 0.2%; lidocaine 1%) |
| | | Calpol Infant Suspension; Calpol Sugar-Free Infant Suspension (packaging change) |
| | | Calpol Six Plus Fastmelts (paracetamol 250mg) |
| | | Acrivastine 8mg |
| | | Bisacodyl 5mg (increased pack size) |

**Source: OTC Bulletin no. 228 September 2004 / MHRA**

**(http://medicines.mhra.gov.uk/inforesources/publications/arm.htm)**

* application not approved

As the table shows, applications for P to GSL switches have greatly outnumbered those for POM to P (by three to one) since the new system to streamline the process was introduced.

The guiding principle of NHS modernisation was the aim of providing services that were best suited to the needs and convenience of patients. Other key aims were to increase self-care and to make better use of health professionals' skills by breaking down traditional inter-professional boundaries. In this context, POM to P switching can be seen as increasing patient autonomy, as well as making more effective use of community pharmacists. Another issue for the NHS is the shortage of doctors and the increasing workload of GPs. POM to P switching could reduce the numbers of GP consultations for common ailments. Increasing the availability of medicines through switching also moves treatment from the NHS into the private sector, as the medicine must be purchased by the patient. It is inevitable that some will view this as privatisation of the NHS.

The cost of OTC medication has been recognised as a barrier to greater self-care, particularly in disadvantaged areas. In response, community pharmacy minor ailments schemes (MAS) have been developed as an NHS service to transfer workload from GPs, as well as to increase choice in England, Scotland and Wales. In Scotland the service is being rolled out across the country. In England the government urged PCTs to consider introducing such a scheme in areas where the cost of OTC medicines was a recognised barrier to their use (Building on the best DH 2003). Some MAS include certain POMs (supplied under Patient Group Direction), as well as OTCs. MAS are considered further in section 1.7: Access to OTC medicines.

POM to P switching can enable access to medicines for an indication that would not qualify for NHS treatment. Simvastatin is the first example, where the argument was made that people should be able to decide for themselves whether they wanted to initiate primary prevention below the level of CHD risk where the NHS would fund treatment. The drivers for POM to P switching and their effects in different countries are reviewed in greater detail elsewhere (Cohen et al 2005).

In its 2003 'Building on the best' paper the government reiterated its commitment to POM to P switching and to the target of 10 switches each year (Building on the best DH 2003). The NHS emphasis on chronic disease management (now termed 'long-term conditions' in the NHS) highlights self-care and suggests that increasing attention will be paid to OTC medicines for long-term conditions. 'Building on the best' listed several therapeutic areas including asthma and migraine for future POM to P switches. In a 2004 conference speech Lord Warner reiterated this commitment (PAGB 2004). Future switches imply the need for education for both the public and for health professionals with the move towards greater self-management of long-term conditions. The extent of public and patient education required here should not be underestimated. The figure below sets out a model of POM to P switching that captures the relative complexity of different switches. The arrow denotes the likely future trend to more switches in new areas of self-care. Quadrant D represents the most complex and demanding switches in terms of education for the public and for professionals, and in relation to the need for effective links between self-care and the NHS.

**Figure 1: Model of complexity of POM to P switching at the time of switch.**

| | | |
|---|---|---|
| **Medicine only available on prescription** | Chloramphenicol eye Drops (2005) | Simvastatin (2004) |
| | **B** ⟶ | **D** |
| | Omeprazole (2004) | |
| Medicine already available OTC | | |
| | **A** | **C** |
| | | Topical hydrocortisone for Eczema (1994) |
| | Current area of self care | New area of self care |

**Key:**

A = Low complexity: medicine already available OTC and indication within existing area of self-care

B = Moderate: existing area of self-care but medicine previously POM (eg chloramphenicol eye drops)

C = Moderate: medicine already available OTC and indication for a new area of self-care

D = High: new area of self-care and medicine previously POM (eg simvastatin)

**Source: Kilby S (2005), Royal Pharmaceutical Society of Great Britain**

Future POM to P switches for long-term conditions will also need greater integration with the wider NHS, for example, management of referrals at the boundary between self-care and NHS care. There is evidence to suggest that a proportion of patients with long-term conditions would appreciate the opportunity for greater self-management with the help and advice of a community pharmacist. Some, however, would choose to continue to use the current medical model. Community pharmacy, under its new contract, is changing and it is anticipated that most premises will have a seated, confidential, consultation area over the next few years. It would be reasonable to measure, for example, PEFR and blood pressure in such a setting. Consequently, switching medicines for the treatment of conditions such as mild to moderate asthma and hypertension would become more feasible. The integration of such a service would require close liaison between community pharmacy and the rest of primary care. Forthcoming developments in NPfIT offer the opportunity to share information across different healthcare settings through the electronic patient record and it is important that OTC medicines for long-term conditions are included. Action is needed now if this is to happen.

The agenda for medicines deregulation is largely driven by the pharmaceutical industry rather than by consideration of needs and priorities from a public health perspective. As the MHRA states: 'Reclassification of a substance normally follows a request from the company which holds a marketing authorisation for it. Requests can however be made by any interested party, such as a professional body, or be initiated by the MHRA' (MHRA 2005). This raises questions about the extent to which OTC medication is, or can be, integrated with wider health strategy. In addition, the short period of time between a consultation being issued for a proposed switch and the launch of the product will inevitably be more challenging for switches of higher complexity. Co-ordinating training for pharmacists and their staff, cascading of local communication at primary care organisation level, formulation of local referral policies and information for the public will be an even greater challenge for the new POM to Ps.

The Royal Pharmaceutical Society, which led a previous multi-stakeholder group on future POM to P switches, is currently planning to build on this work with stakeholders from 2005. Work on integration of OTC medication into the wider NHS is needed as part of these developments.

## 1.6 Doctors' attitudes to OTC medication

Doctors are an important influence on OTC use in several ways. They may recommend (or advise against) certain medicines, and prescribe medicines that are available OTC.

There is evidence that the attitudes of British GPs towards OTC availability of medicines have become more positive over time (table 6). Around the time of early POM to P moves in the 1980s GPs showed a cautious approach to potential switches (Morley et al 1983), but more recent surveys show a majority of GPs in favour of many potential switches.

**Table 6: Level of GP agreement to potential POM to P switches**

| | Morley et al 1983 | Spencer 1992 | Erwin & Britten 1996 | Bayliss & Rutter 2004 |
|---|---|---|---|---|
| Topical hydrocortisone | 26% | - | Deregulated | 1994 |
| Steroid-containing suppositories for haemorrhoids | 50% | - | | |
| Chlorampenicol eye drops | 34% | 52% | 67% | 80% |
| Co-dydramol tablets | 41% | 87% | 87% | 87% |
| Topical antibiotics | 18% | 30% | 40% | 94% |
| Trimethoprim | - | 35% | 55% | 66% |
| Triptans | - | - | - | 61% |
| Thiazide diuretics for hypertension | - | - | - | 13% |

The authors of the most recent study of GP attitudes towards POM to P switches concluded that their findings 'suggest that GPs agree to the deregulation of medicines used to treat acute illness but are opposed to those used in chronic conditions' (Bayliss and Rutter 2004). The reasons for this shift in opinion have not been formally researched but may include acceptance of a now established policy, perceived lack of problems with previous switches, and their own increasing workload. Consideration of the trend shown over the last two decades indicates that GPs' views may in time become more positive towards OTC treatment for long-term conditions. A survey of Finnish doctors, for example, found that attitudes were moderately positive, but 'more reserved towards those drugs only recently given OTC status' (Sihvo et al 1999).

Research has shown that GPs' rates of recommending OTC treatment ranged from 2.3 per cent to 37.5 per cent of consultations, and that this was usually in addition to, rather than instead of, giving a prescription (Bradley 1996). The main reason GPs gave for recommending OTC medicines was that they were cheaper for some patients. Very few of these recommendations were for medicines that had switched from POM to P. These findings suggest that doctors are reluctant to advise use of an OTC medicine instead of prescribing a treatment. A key reason for this was that NHS terms of service required the doctor to give a prescription where they believed a medicine to be necessary. Another reason may be the extent of GPs' knowledge about the medicines and products available OTC. There is little published research on this subject, but there is some evidence that GPs may not be aware of the restrictions on use of certain medicines (Rogers et al 2004). Undergraduate medical education is generally viewed as including relatively little teaching on medicines and prescribing, so it seems unlikely that OTC medicines are extensively covered.

We found only one published paper, from the US, addressing teaching about OTC medicines in medical schools (Henley and Wenzel-Wamhoff 2000).

The difficulty, once a patient has made an appointment and travelled to the surgery, of suggesting to them that they should go and buy a medicine instead was also frequently cited (Bradley 1996). Medical endorsement of OTC treatment is likely to be a powerful factor influencing patients' behaviour. These findings suggest that education campaigns for the public that are clearly endorsed by doctors are likely to be needed if behaviour is to change. The 'self-care aware consultation' currently being tested could also make an important contribution (Adcock H 2004).

The extent to which doctors prescribe medicines where there is an available OTC treatment has been the subject of few studies. A UK analysis found that an increase in the number of OTC items prescribed corresponded to greater levels of prepayment or exemption among patients registered with the GP practice (Baines and Whynes 1997). A US study found that 10 per cent of medicines prescribed were available OTC and that OTC/POM ratios were highest in family practice, internal medicine, obstetrics/gynaecology and paediatrics (Pradel et al 1999). Such data are difficult to interpret and have been subject to some unrealistic conclusions, for example, that ideally patients would be expected to buy treatments available OTC. In the USA the OTC availability of second generation antihistamine loratadine led some healthcare providers to remove it from their formulary or to increase co-payments to encourage people to purchase it OTC instead (Cohen et al 2005). A UK study found that around 40 per cent of respondents agreed that 'I sometimes cannot afford to buy all the medicines I would like to buy myself without prescription' (Bradley et al 1998). Recognition that cost is a reason why some people choose to consult their GP rather than self-treat led to the development and spread of community pharmacy NHS Minor Ailment Schemes as a means of transferring workload away from GPs (see Access to OTC medicines).

## 1.7 Access to OTC medicines

OTC medicines are available from both public and private sector sources. The methods of access provide relatively higher or lower levels of control over their use (figure 2).

**Figure 2: Access to OTC medicines**

*Less control over use* ————————————————→ *More control over use*

| 'Off-the-shelf' | 'Behind-the-counter' | 'In the dispensary' |
|---|---|---|
| GSL medicines | P medicines | POM medicines |
| | | Patient Group Directions |

Community Pharmacy NHS Minor Ailment Schemes

NHS Access includes prescriptions (doctors, nurses, dentists, pharmacists), Patient Group Directions (PGDs) and NHS community pharmacy MAS. The formularies for independent nurse prescribing (INPF) and extended nurse prescribing (ENPF) enable nurses to prescribe for a wide range of minor ailments. PGDs have been used to widen availability of certain POM medicines. Examples in community pharmacy include chloramphenicol eye drops for infective conjunctivitis and trimethoprim for uncomplicated urinary tract infection. At the time of writing the MHRA was consulting on the scope and content of pharmacist independent prescribing. The implementation of independent prescribing by pharmacists may lead to opportunities for pharmacists to prescribe some medicines for common illnesses that are currently POM.

---

**Community pharmacy NHS Minor Ailment Schemes**

The first community pharmacy NHS MAS was introduced in Sefton in 1997 and provided certain medicines for specified minor ailments free of charge to people who were exempt from NHS prescription charges. By late 2004, schemes were available in an estimated 100 PCTs in England, with schemes also in Scotland and Wales and government policy was supporting their provision targeted in disadvantaged areas (Building on the best 2003). The schemes have a locally agreed list of ailments to be treated and treatments are supplied based on a local formulary. They have been shown to be used by people who would otherwise have seen their GP and to be well received by the public (Hassell et al 2001; Blenkinsopp and Noyce 2002; Walker et al 2003). Some incorporate the use of PGDs to manage additional conditions such as infective conjunctivitis, impetigo and urinary tract infections. A toolkit for PCTs to support commissioning of MAS was produced in 2004 (National Pharmaceutical Association 2004).

---

Private sector availability includes community pharmacies, general retail outlets (newsagents, garage forecourt shops, supermarkets) and the internet. Professional advice is available on some internet-based pharmacy sites, but such support is not available to those purchasing OTC medicines from non-pharmacy outlets.

# 2. Patient/user perspectives

Relatively little is known about what the public thinks about OTC medication for long-term conditions, but there is a body of literature about the use of OTC medicines for the management of minor illness. It will become increasingly important to carry out research in this area; the perceived inequity of access to medicines between different groups of people with long-term conditions and those in different income groups will influence readiness to access OTC medicines for an increasingly wide range of conditions. The increasing use of the internet to obtain medicines of all kinds, but especially POMs, indicates an eagerness on the part of some patients/users to gain more convenient access to medicines with fewer or no controls exerted by either doctors or pharmacists. There is no published research to show the knowledge and experience of this group of medicine purchasers. This, among other things, indicates a need for education of the public about the benefits of getting professional advice and input into their medicine taking and the potential risks of unsupervised medicine consumption.

## 2.1 Decision making about OTC medicines

It is required that sales of medicines in the P category are supervised by a pharmacist. In practice, community pharmacies have a written protocol that sets out how staff will deal with OTC medicine sales. The acceptability of this concept with the public is debatable. Although most consumers in one UK study had a degree of awareness of why pharmacy staff might require information, almost two thirds had expected to make their most recent purchase without being questioned (Morris et al 1997). A Canadian study of consumers purchasing medicines in pharmacies without asking for advice found that over 90 per cent had used the product before or had received advice elsewhere about what to purchase (Taylor 1994). These findings indicate that many people buying medicines in a pharmacy may not consider it the legitimate business of pharmacy staff to ask what they may view as 'personal' questions about why the medicine was needed. This creates a potential conflict between the public health role of community pharmacy staff and the nature of consumer autonomy in purchasing a medicine. One way for pharmacists to deal with this potential dissonance is to differentiate between 'novice' and 'expert' users of OTC medicines. This is an area that the Royal Pharmaceutical Society needs to consider, with the involvement of medicine users, not only in its work on future POM to P switches but also more widely in relation to OTC medicines.

There is some evidence from the UK (Bissell et al 2001) and the USA (Roumie and Griffin 2004) that members of the public regard OTC medicines as inherently 'weaker' than prescription medicines. OTC status in itself may lead to a perception that the medicine cannot be harmful, for example, 40 per cent of people in a US study believed that OTC medicines were 'too weak to cause any real harm' (Roumie and Griffin 2004). That doses of medicines switched from POM to P may be lower than those used on prescription is likely to reinforce such beliefs, even though evidence on effectiveness of the lower dose for OTC medications will have been considered in the regulatory process.

User awareness of active ingredients in OTC medicines is an important safety issue and labelling is key, particularly for combination products. One US study found that more than 60 per cent of older people could not identify the active ingredient in their brand of pain relief, leading to a call for improved labelling of OTC analgesics and enhanced education for both healthcare providers and patients (Roumie and Griffin 2004).

The information accompanying the medicine and how that information is presented is a factor in how safely the medicine is used. Information leaflets inside medicine packages need further attention, in particular they need to describe in more detail the rationale for the medicine's use, its benefits, and when to consult a doctor and pharmacist. Some of the current standard wording, for example, 'If symptoms persist, consult your doctor' is too non-specific to be helpful.

As medicines for longer term use are re-categorised as OTC there will need to be information to the effect that the medicine should be taken long-term and the need for medical and pharmaceutical input must be stressed in both leaflet and label. The MHRA is working on implementation of user testing for manufacturers' Patient Information Leaflets (PILs) for both prescription and OTC medicines, incorporating evidence on the presentation of benefits and risks. Labelling is a critical factor in successful self-selection of GSL medicines as well as safe use of both GSLs and Ps. User testing of package labels is also needed.

The extent to which the use of OTC medicine either substitutes for, or simply delays, consultation with a health professional is difficult to determine. A US study following the POM to P switch of omeprazole found that 26 per cent of subjects who purchased OTC omeprazole had contact with a physician about their heartburn during the following three months (Fendrick et al 2004). These data are difficult to interpret without knowing the reasons why these patients chose to consult.

## 2.2 Influences on OTC use

Unlike prescription products OTC medicines can be advertised directly to the public. While there is a formal system in place to approve the content of advertisements, their content can nonetheless appear to overstate benefits, and omit mentioning other points such as price (Rallapalli and Smith 1994). This will inevitably influence purchasers in favour of the product. A study from the USA concluded that the advertisements lacked the information necessary for consumers to make informed choices (Sansgiry et al 1999). There is no similar published research on UK advertisements for OTC medicines.

The extent, however, to which doctors and patients discuss OTC treatments is less clear. In a US study 58 per cent of patients discussed OTC medicines with their doctors (Sleath 2001). The participating patients were those attending primary care consultations and so had the opportunity for such discussion. Doctors asked questions about OTC medication in 37 per cent of consultations. The authors concluded that physician-patient communication about OTC medications should be encouraged so that the patient becomes a collaborative partner in medication management. Health professionals may or may not perceive a need to know what OTC medicines patients are taking. While this may change if patient-held records, or smart cards are introduced, we know little about how patients themselves might view discussion with health professionals about self-medication. Little is known about the extent to which prescribers (medical, nursing or pharmacist) routinely enquire about OTC medicines use in their consultations with patients. In one UK study 45 per cent of people consulting their GP reported using OTC medicines in the previous week, but only 13 per cent were asked about this by the doctor (Urquhart et al 2004). Patients were generally positive about the idea that doctors might enquire about prior OTC use, as well as doctors making OTC recommendations (Bradley 1998) but there is also evidence that patients feel inhibited from volunteering information about prior treatment with OTCs (Stevenson et al 2003).

Branstad *et al* studied the effects of OTC availability of topical hydrocortisone (via pharmacy-only sales) in Sweden (Branstad et al 1994). Magazine articles were found to be the most frequently cited source of information around the time of the switch. Six years after the switch, however, pharmacy staff and nurses had become the most important sources. Research suggests that doctors may be more highly rated than pharmacists as sources of information about OTC medicines (Lefterova and Getov 2004, Gore and Madhavan 1993).

## 2.3 Older people and OTC medicines

Polypharmacy of prescribed medicines is more prevalent among older people and increases the potential for drug interactions when OTC medicines are used. Older people's consultations with health professionals often omit discussions of OTC medicines, and there have been calls for medication histories to include documentation of any OTC medicines taken (Barnett et al 2000). In the UK, changes in NHS policy have led to more frequent reviews of patients' medicines and it is important that these take OTC medicines into account.

Older people were found to request help from the pharmacist more often than young adults in one US study and were also more likely to read OTC labels 'completely' (Sansgiry and Cady 1996).

## 2.4 Children and OTC medicines

Parents' use of medicines to treat their children's illnesses has been examined in several studies (see, for example, McIntyre et al 2003; Birchley and Conroy 2002). A qualitative study in the UK explored in depth how parents made decisions in relation to OTC medicines (Birchley and Conroy 2002). The decision about whether to seek advice was based on severity of symptoms and parental experience. OTC medicines were viewed as costly by 16 of the 25 participants, but convenience, accessibility and choice were factors that led to OTC purchases. The researchers recommended that healthcare professionals should remember and explore the use of OTC medicine use when children present for treatment.

## 2.5 Compliance with OTC medicines

Compared to decision making about prescribed medicines, agreement between the patient and prescriber is likely when seeking advice about OTC medicines since the user is, by definition, making the choice to purchase and use the treatment. It might, therefore, be expected that compliance would also be higher. However, we found no research evidence to support or refute this. If OTC medicines are to be used for long-term conditions then compliance could become an issue and further research is needed to clarify this, and the potential role of the pharmacist in monitoring treatment.

Compliance with the intended use of OTC medicines is another important aspect. A large US study of users of OTC omeprazole found that consumers accurately self-selected the treatment and almost all complied with the recommended maximum self-treatment period of 14 days (Fendrick et al 2004). Another US study which simulated OTC availability of lovastatin found that most participants appropriately self-selected OTC statin therapy with a small proportion who used the statin, but needed more intensive statin therapy or faced a potential drug-to-drug interaction (Brass 2004).

# 3. Balance of benefits and risks

OTC medicines have traditionally always been available from community pharmacies and their place in healthcare is widely recognised, particularly for treating what are seen as minor ailments or self-limiting disease. Most recently, reflecting the increasing numbers of effective drugs available, the range of OTC medicines has also increased through the process of deregulation already described. The rationale for the deregulation of medicines is multifactorial and includes benefits to the NHS and the industry, as well as increased convenience and autonomy for patients (Brass 2001). Any risks of deregulation, however, must be balanced against these benefits in order to be confident that the deregulation has been in the overall public interest. Thus, patient safety is a major concern and an issue that should be addressed on a case-by-case basis depending on the drug in question.

The criteria for decisions about POM to P deregulation (discussed earlier in this report) can be regarded as the safety framework within which drugs should **not** be made freely available to the public. They specify the circumstances where unregulated use could pose more risk than benefit. The framework is now used in this section as a basis for considering the risks and benefits of OTC medicines in general. In summary, these are that a drug should remain a POM if any of the following apply:

- the need for medical supervision to monitor adverse events or ensure correct diagnosis
- the risk of incorrect use leading to danger to health (eg misuse)
- the need for further investigation of the drug
- parenteral administration.

Despite their apparent clarity, each of the four criteria is subject to a degree of interpretation. Within the current armamentarium of drugs either already 'switched' or currently undergoing consultation for switching there are examples which break each of these rules. For example, of the well-established medicines available OTC, paracetamol is not safe in overdose, GTN[3] is not for a minor illness or self-limiting condition and its use should be informed by an accurate diagnosis, and many traditional painkillers and some anti-diarrhoeals contain opioids such as codeine or morphine which can be abused. Apparent anomalies within more newly deregulated OTCs are considered in more detail in the following sections.

## 3.1 Risk of adverse events

All pharmacologically active substances will have a main 'intended' effect and other effects known as 'side effects'. Side effects may be beneficial in their own right, cause a minor inconvenience, or pose a serious threat to health. OTC drugs are no exception.

Adverse events associated with a drug can either be potentially predictable based on pharmacological principles, or idiosyncratic and therefore unexpected. There might also be an increase in a common event, which may not immediately be linked to drug use.

---

[3] Glyceryl trinitrate.

The unexpected are almost always rare events, may arise as a direct result of the action of the drug *per se,* or its interaction with other drugs. In retrospect they might have been predictable as with the COX-2 selective NSAIDs.[4] By virtue of their rarity, they are increasingly likely to be identified as volume of usage increases. Some adverse events can be fatal.

When a new medicine is proposed for deregulation its current safety profile, as a prescription-only medicine, is one of the key data sources used to inform decision making. At that point, however, the above noted rare events may not be apparent and continued systematic pharmacovigilance is important to monitor events as usage increases as a result of OTC availability. Reassessment of status as an OTC may also be necessary as is illustrated by the example below.

One of the first medicines to be deregulated was the second-generation non-sedating antihistamine terfenadine. It is a good example of a well-used drug which caused an idiosyncratic adverse event, which was only identified after widespread use. It was deregulated in 1984, and in 1992 was formally linked to serious and sometimes fatal cardiac arrhythmias. This occurred when terfenadine was taken by patients with cardiac or hepatic disease, in overdose, or with drugs with which it interacted (eg ketoconazole), or certain food stuffs (eg grapefruit juice) (Anonymous 1997, Committee for Safety of Medicines and Medicines Control Agency 1992). The product was first restored to prescription-only use (1997), but soon removed completely from UK availability.

Perhaps more unexpected have been the serious interactions between the herbal preparation St John's Wort (hypericum perforatum) and some commonly prescribed drugs, including warfarin, ciclosporin, oral contraceptives, digoxin, theophylline, and selective serotonin reuptake inhibitors. Reduced blood concentrations of these drugs result from the enzyme inducing properties of St John's Wort. Although theoretically predictable, the herbal classification of the product means that there are limited regulatory mechanisms in the UK to control its distribution and use. Awareness of the specific problem with St John's Wort has been raised through official letters from the Committee on Safety of Medicines to pharmacists and doctors (Committee on Safety of Medicines 2000). In Ireland certain herbal remedies such as St John's Wort have relatively recently been

---

[4] COX-2 selective NSAIDs are associated with increased risk of cardiovascular events and several have now been withdrawn or are subject to 'caution in use' advice (Committee on Safety of Medicines 2004). These selective NSAIDs were associated with reduced gastro intestinal effects compared to non- selective NSAIDs because of the limited inhibition of COX-1 which has a gastro protective effect. However inhibition of COX-1 is also related to reduced blood clot formation. This is the rationale for people to take daily low dose aspirin, and one explanation for the increased cardiovascular risk of the COX-2 drugs (Davies and Jamali 2004).

[5] 'On the basis of the data available, the Committee on Safety of Medicines (CSM) has reached the provisional view that the possible therapeutic benefits of medicinal products containing the herbal ingredient kava-kava (piper methysticum) can not be considered to outweigh the safety risks. Kava-kava is considered to have the potential to cause hepatotoxicity which may be serious. The level of risk is not known but is likely to be rare at normal doses. The mechanism of toxicity is not understood and there are no clear predictors of toxicity' CEM/CMO/2002/10

reclassified as POM, although this is reported to have been an unpopular move with the public. A further example of a safety issue with a herbal product is kava-kava[5] (Breckenridge 2002). Of general concern is the fact that the 'herbal' label seems to be associated by the public with safety due to its 'natural' content, resulting in a lack of recognition from both the public and professionals of the potential potency of the products.

Some side effects may be predictable such as the increased risk of gastro-intestinal bleeding from the use of NSAIDs. Although there is some evidence that ibuprofen is as safe as paracetamol when used at OTC doses, and for short duration (Moore et al 1999) it cannot always be assumed that OTC drug users will adhere to the licensing restrictions. In a small Scottish study (Sinclair et al 2001, Sinclair et al 2000), purchasers of ibuprofen were followed up over six months. Subjects reported that they were using OTC ibuprofen for long-term conditions, and over extended periods of time (for example more than 13 weeks). More significantly, just under 10 per cent took doses above those recommended for OTC use, and some even above the recommended prescribed dose. Small numbers also took ibuprofen when they had an active or past history of peptic ulcer, or asthma, both of which are contra-indicated co-morbidities. Patient follow up indicated an increased incidence of GI events. However, the key finding is that it cannot be assumed that all OTC medicine users will adhere to the recommended dosage regimes on which predicted safety is based. Improved labelling, patient education and support might be ways to overcome these problems while maintaining the advantages of OTC availability.

The examples given above illustrate the need to be alert to the potential for 'safe' OTC drugs to cause unexpected problems, either when used on their own or in combination with other prescribed products. Formal mechanisms should be in place to support this and are discussed further in section 5, Information and communication.

## 3.2 Impact of OTC medication on diagnosis

Correct diagnosis is essential in recommending safe and appropriate treatment, and this is no less so for OTC medicines than for prescribed medicines. The corollary is that incorrect diagnosis could result in inappropriate management and increased risk. The practicalities and limitations of a diagnostic consultation OTC are addressed in the next section; here we will consider the sequelae of misdiagnosis from a safety perspective.

There are two scenarios that should be avoided. One is the possibility that the use of the OTC drug could mask the symptoms of a serious disease, thus delaying diagnosis and potentially worsening prognosis. The other is that a drug might be used ineffectively, so that the patient has been exposed to unnecessary costs and risks of a drug with no likelihood of any benefit. Either of these scenarios would run counter to the criterion of safe and appropriate treatment.

While pain killers could always be considered to be in the first category, for example being used to treat prolonged and severe headaches which might have been due to sinister causes, this has not in fact been raised as a reason for restricting their availability, possibly because aspirin and paracetamol have long been regarded as established OTC analgesics. However, when a new category of drug was considered for switching, as was the case with the H2 blockers, there were widely expressed concerns that their use could lead to the masking of symptoms of gastric cancer. Thus, guidelines were quickly developed (Bond and Grimshaw 1994) to aid pharmacy staff in their differential diagnosis of epigastric pain. To the best of our knowledge there have been no reports or studies published since the deregulation of H2 antagonists, which have given credibility to the aforementioned theoretical concerns.

While symptomatic treatments are most likely to cause concern about delaying diagnosis, misdiagnosis and unnecessary treatment are more likely for compounds with a specific targeted action. An example of a medicine in this category is the vaginal imidazoles, first deregulated in 1997, for the specific treatment of vaginal candidiasis (thrush). Guidance was developed for pharmacists to aid in their diagnosis and management of thrush (Watson and Bond 2003). While the risk of missing other more serious causes of similar symptoms is less clear than for the H2 blockers, the symptom based diagnostic criteria for candida have both poor specificity and sensitivity (Anderson et al 2004). Other more serious vaginal conditions can mimic the symptoms, and if untreated can result in prolonged unnecessary discomfort to the patient. Mechanisms such as self-administered diagnostic swabs for subsequent mycological culture may be a future way to inform diagnosis and management OTC. Self-administered tampons to detect sexually transmitted diseases (Wiesenfeld et al 2001) are already available and there is a theoretical possibility of developing such a test for the diagnosis of candidiasis.

## 3.3 Misuse

Misuse of OTC drugs is of concern in a minority of users, as this next section will illustrate. The potential for misuse of OTC drugs has also been the subject of recent media stories. It is important that healthcare professionals and the public are aware of these issues and work in partnership to reduce them.

Although clear, written, and often verbal guidance on OTC medicines is given, patients may deliberately or inadvertently take the medicine differently from the labelled instructions and recommendations. Deliberate misuse would include the taking of a drug purely for recreational effect (eg an opioid, or an antihistamine), or exceeding the recommended OTC dose, or duration of treatment, to experience enhanced medicinal effects (eg an analgesic or a sleep aid). Inadvertent misuse could include long-term regular use of a drug with increased risk of developing side effects, (for example NSAID use). While products sold from pharmacies will be subject to supervision from the pharmacist, who may use a variety of protocols to maximise benefit and minimise harm to patients, this is not the case for products sold from general retail outlets. Pharmacists' Code of Ethics requires that, 'pharmacists and their staff must be aware of the abuse potential of certain OTC products and should not supply where there are reasonable grounds for suspecting misuse' (RPSGB 2004).

While reasonable grounds are not defined within the Code, examples might be that customers were obviously purchasing quantities in excess of those required under a standard dosing schedule, or regular purchase without apparent clinical indications for using the drug.

Research shows that community pharmacists are concerned about possible misuse of OTC medicines and use a variety of strategies to detect and prevent this, including registers of use, refusing sales (in line with their Code of Ethics), removing certain products from display or not stocking them at all (Pates et al 2002, Hughes et al 1999). Work conducted in Scotland in 1995 and 2000 (Matheson et al 2002) found that over two thirds of community pharmacists reported having suspicions of the misuse of OTC medicines, confirming an earlier small survey in Wales (Pates et al 2002). This was particularly the case in urban areas. Four broad categories of products were mentioned: antihistamines, opioids, mild stimulants, and laxatives. Throughout Scotland, the misuse of antihistamine-containing products was suspected by more than half of all community pharmacists: this could be excessive use (outside the recommended dosage) for sleep disturbances or to mask other drug dependence. There was a reduction in the suspected misuse of codeine linctus across the two surveys, although not other codeine containing products. Similarly, sleep aids and codeine containing analgesics were products found to generate the most concern in another UK study (Phelan et al 2003). An international survey of strategies used and suggested by community pharmacists to reduce misuse of OTC sleep aids identified some key areas. These included improving access to current information, improved staff training, and addressing the issues of OTC sales from non-pharmacy outlets and over the internet (McBride et al 2003). Pharmacists must, therefore, continue to be vigilant regarding the potential for inappropriate or excessive consumption or use of these medicines, in line with their Code of Ethics.

Drugs with a serious potential for addiction are covered by the Misuse of Drugs Act, and their distribution controlled carefully through formal prescribing. Small doses of controlled drugs, such as dihydrocodeine, codeine and morphine are, however, still allowable OTC as components of compound preparations. There are still several proprietary brands of antidiarrhoeals for example, which contain small amounts of morphine, and cough remedies which contain codeine. Codeine and dihydrocodeine are constituents of some OTC analgesics, in combination with aspirin, paracetamol or ibuprofen. Pharmacists are reported to be concerned about drug misusers attempting to purchase codeine-containing analgesics (Pates et al 2002, Hughes et al 1999).

There has been some research specifically into the overuse of sleep aids. First generation antihistamines (FGAs) including diphenydramine and promethazine are available over the counter in several countries as sleep aids. Such products may be inadvertently misused by people whose sleep disorder is other than a temporary problem. They may also be deliberately misused by people dependent on other medicines. A UK study found that some users had been taking the sleep aid for longer than the recommended time (Phelan et al 2003). Usage of antihistamine sleep aids in the USA is higher than that of benzodiazepines and a US study of people with sleep problems found that 6.4 per cent of men and 11.4 per cent of women reported using OTC sleep aids

(Pillitteri et al 1994). The percentages of men and women reporting using alcohol to help them sleep were higher, at 23.4 per cent and 10.9 per cent. Just over a quarter of people aged over 60 in a Canadian survey of patients during hospital or pharmacy visits had used an OTC sleep aid within the last year (Sproule et al 1999). The same study found that 19 per cent of people who reported using a sleep aid cited paracetamol and 13 per cent alcohol.

Sleep aids and analgesics containing opioids may also be deliberately misused by people dependent on other medicines, but there is probably most concern about inadvertent dependence on such products developing following prolonged use. For example, the long-term use of analgesics in the treatment of chronic daily headache can lead to inadvertent dependence and rebound headache on withdrawal. This applies to both OTC and prescribed analgesics.

There are no epidemiological data to enable reliable estimates of incidence or prevalence of OTC medicine misuse. A support group for people dependent on OTC medicines, Over Count, estimated that 30,000 people might be affected by such dependence in Great Britain (Grieve D 2004). The lack of data on usage of OTC analgesics across the population of users, however, means it is impossible to support or refute this estimate. This again supports the need for a systematic approach to recording use of OTC medicines and their pharmacovigilance.

The individual case histories collected by Over Count do indicate that some users of OTC analgesics whose symptoms are not controlled within the parameters of recommended timescale and dose need support in obtaining further information and advice. Over Count has advocated that product labelling should warn of the possibility of dependence. Others have argued, however, that such labelling would be counter-productive (for example, deterring use by people who might benefit) and could encourage misuse (Adcock H 2001). Health professionals need to be aware of the small possibility of dependence on OTC medicines and of what support patients might need to stop using the medicine.

In summary, the important issue is probably whether misuse is deliberate or inadvertent. It is necessary to balance the important benefits of the OTC availability of effective treatments, to both the NHS and the majority of the population, against the risk of misuse. The efforts of regulators and healthcare professionals should go into ensuring that inadvertent misuse is avoided and that deliberate misuse (ie those taking a drug for recreational effect or enhanced medicinal effects) is identified early and dealt with appropriately.

## 3.4 Further investigation required

As described, all newly marketed drugs are classified as a POM. This means that while a new drug entity is still being monitored closely it is unlikely to be available OTC, and thus the third criterion for retaining POM status 'further investigation required' is less likely to apply to OTC medicines than the two previously discussed (the need for supervision because of issues of adverse events or diagnosis, and the potential for incorrect usage [misuse]). Once circumstances change however, new investigations might be required to confirm OTC safety, and hence appropriateness of OTC availability of a drug. This should mean that the product would revert to POM status for this period, as happened when suspicions of carcinogenicity were associated with the head lice treatment carbaryl (Anonymous 1995).

## 3.5 Parenteral use

The least contentious category might be parenteral use and few would be likely to advocate OTC injectables in the current climate. However, there is an ongoing POM to P consultation for Water for Injection to allow drug misusers to purchase this from accredited needle exchanges and thus reduce the individual and societal harm associated with the injection of drugs. Once such precedents are set, then it would theoretically be easier for other 'harmless' injectables to be made available OTC, for selected groups, for example those for use in life-saving circumstances such as adrenaline for anaphylactic shock.

## 3.6 Availability versus control

The above paragraphs have considered the potential risks associated with OTC medication against the background of the regulatory framework that allows their use. It has also illustrated the ill-defined nature of these regulations and the need for their careful interpretation to achieve the responsible use of medicines. The POM legislation imposes controls on the supply of medicines such that the risks can be monitored by a professional to the benefit of the patient taking the drug. There is ongoing debate about the extent to which control should be relinquished completely at the point of deregulation. In the UK there are three categories of medicines classification (see earlier). The first tier after the POM is the P. In this category, the pharmacist and his/her staff have a professional responsibility to ensure the safe and effective supply and use of medicines (Royal Pharmaceutical Society of Great Britain 2004), which requires a degree of intervention, and may result in refusal to supply a requested product. Slow initial sales of the then newly deregulated H2 blockers were attributed to the reluctance of pharmacists to promote their sale. It has been suggested that if pharmacists take on this gatekeeper role, it is merely replacing the traditional paternalistic medical prescriber with a pharmacist and is not widening access to medicines or empowering the public (Prayle and Brazier 1998). This negative attitude however ignores the increased accessibility and convenience of accessing medicines directly from a retail outlet, or the supportive, rather than prescriptive role of the pharmacist in self-care. Thus, the key principle of wider access to medicines is maintained, while including an element of risk management.

In contrast, in the USA there is no intermediate category of drug classification and the range of OTC products is generally more limited than in the UK, although there are some anomalies (for example, topical antibiotics are available OTC in the USA). Conversely, in Australia and New Zealand there is a fourth category of pharmacist-only medicines, which requires the personal involvement of the pharmacist in every sale. This has empowered the pharmacist to ask more searching questions at the point of sale.

An alternative to amendments to the actual classification of a medicine is a change to the specific details of the OTC licence. When there were widespread concerns about the numbers of fatalities attributed to paracetamol overdose for example, the response was not to revert to POM status, but to limit the OTC pack size, and total quantity which could be sold OTC. There were initial concerns that this move would not be sufficient to address the problem. Since the change, the number of paracetamol associated fatalities appears to have been reduced, although a recent paper reminds us that without a control group the true cause of this trend is unknown (Morgan et al 2005). An alternative approach adopted in the USA was to add methionine to the paracetamol (ie the antidote which is harmless) but that 'admits' there is a problem with its toxicity.

Conversely, as confidence in the safe and appropriate use of deregulated products is acquired, then the OTC indications can become extended, for example the prophylactic use of H2 blockers to protect against 'over indulgence'. The dosage available might also be increased. For example, the first nicotine replacement product to be deregulated was the 2mg chewing gum, but since then there has been subsequent availability of a 4mg strength, as well as other formulations such as patches and inhalators. Further, in the UK, complete deregulation from P to GSL status is the ultimate natural progression when there is confidence in the drug's safety in wider use. While truly achieving maximum public accessibility and convenience, this further reduces the chance of any health professional input. Some of the disadvantages of this are discussed in the next section.

# 4. Role of professionals

## 4.1 Pharmacists and their staff

The deregulation of medicines from POM is normally to P as a first step, transferring the responsibility for appropriate supply from the doctor to the pharmacist and his/her staff. The RPSGB, as noted already, has specific sections in their Code of Ethics (Royal Pharmaceutical Society of Great Britain 2004) to ensure that this responsibility is adequately delivered, and includes five specific types of supply: advice for treatment, requests for a named product, personal involvement of the pharmacist 'when necessary', procedures to ensure that specific groups (eg the young or the elderly) receive particular care, and procedures for specific medicines such as those that have recently become available without prescription.

Evidence from observational and patient studies shows that most OTC sales of medicines are dealt with by medicine counter assistants (MCAs) (Watson and Bond 2004; Emmerton and Shaw 2002). The sale of OTC medicines is an increasingly important clinical role and the RPSGB has recognised the need to ensure that the counter assistants managing the majority of these transactions are appropriately trained to give basic advice and to know when to seek input from their supervisory pharmacist. As a result, it became mandatory in 1996 for all assistants involved in the role of medicines to be trained to NVQ level 2 (Anonymous 1994a), and in 1995 for all pharmacies to have in place protocols for the sale of OTC medicines (Anonymous 1994b, 1994c). Most recently, the RPSGB has moved to register and regulate all pharmacy technicians from 2005; while not all MCAs will immediately register as technicians, which requires a higher level of training than NVQ2, this will inevitably become a goal for them to work towards.

OTC product choice, as with most prescribing decisions, was historically based on experience and serendipitous feedback from customers. In an era of evidence-based medicine, and with increasingly potent medicines now available OTC, it is important that OTC sales are conducted in line with the best evidence. Reflecting this objective, guidelines have been produced covering topics such as dyspepsia and constipation (Matheson and Bond 1995, Bond and Grimshaw 1994). They have been well received by pharmacists. As the general understanding of the need to assess the quality of evidence has increased, pharmacy guidelines for OTC medicines have increasingly become more robust (Bousquet et al 2004) and some have been developed on the basis of recognised systematic reviews, such as one for the treatment of vaginal thrush (Watson et al 2003).

As with other areas of healthcare, implementing such evidence-based guidelines is key to their successful impact on health outcomes. An RCT comparing conventional continuing education workshops with educational outreach and unsupported mailings showed no difference between the groups in the outcome of appropriate supply of vaginal imidazoles, as assessed by role playing actors (Watson et al 2002). Alongside the conventional RCT, a Theory of Planned Behaviour (TPB) survey indicated other factors than clinical knowledge and intention to supply were acting as barriers (Walker et al 2003). Further work is ongoing but early observational studies and interviews indicate that failure to communicate effectively with customers, and hence failure to elicit all the necessary information are major shortcomings. Interestingly, the main concerns of medicines counter assistants are for the safety of the supply and their liability (Watson and Bond 2004). Contrary to popular belief there is little commercial pressure to sell a patient a product unless its supply is deemed appropriate. Secondary analyses of the RCT described above demonstrated that the higher the number of information items exchanged in the OTC transaction, the greater was the likelihood of an appropriate outcome (Watson personal communication 2005; paper submitted).

The increased availability of OTC medicines, as described, is achieved by a range of supply routes. Although primarily through deregulation and private purchases, other mechanisms include direct supply. The wider access to medicines through deregulation to P sale has been criticised as it widens the health inequality gap. Those patients normally exempt from prescription charges would have little incentive to purchase the same drugs OTC, often in more limited quantities. Research has shown that people who could self-medicate are unwilling to do so for financial reasons (Hassell et al 1999: Payne et al 1998, Schafheutle et al 1996). This results in unnecessary medical consultations, solely for the purpose of procuring a drug. In a move to overcome this, 'direct supply' arrangements have been successfully piloted and evaluated (Whittington et al 2001). In such schemes, patients normally exempt from the prescription levy can receive a limited range of drugs direct from their community pharmacist, within the NHS. Examples of other schemes include treatments for head lice (Anonymous 2001), smoking cessation (Anonymous 2002) and emergency hormonal contraception (Anonymous 2000). The new community pharmacy contract recently negotiated in England and Scotland includes provision for this supply to become a core pharmacy service in Scotland and locally-commissioned in England.

## 4.2 General practitioners

There are several points in the medical consultation at which the GP should be aware of OTC medicines. This will become increasingly so as the range and potency of OTC medicines increases.

Initially, when a patient presents and a history is taken, key questions from the GP should include an enquiry into OTC use. An OTC medicine might be responsible for the presenting symptoms, such as constipation from an opioid analgesic, or exacerbated asthma or peptic ulcer after ibuprofen use. The Scottish survey referred to previously (Sinclair et al 2001, 2000) included patients' reports of these sorts of events. One woman taking ibuprofen for example, reported that she went to the GP with increased epigastric pain and was prescribed a PPI without any enquiry into concomitant medication use.

Knowledge of previous use of an OTC medicine, and its effect, will also be an important diagnostic tool, and inform subsequent medical prescribing. A significant number of patients are prescribed preparations including the same drug, or a therapeutic equivalent of a drug they are taking OTC. This OTC use might be prior to the initial consultation, or subsequent to it if the prescribed medication is less effective than required. A population based Scottish survey of OTC analgesic use reported that 37 per cent of respondents had used a non-prescription analgesic in the previous two weeks, accounting for 59 per cent of all non-prescription medicines used. There was evidence of possible inappropriate use of non-prescription analgesics including use of multiple analgesics, use by individuals self-reporting conditions associated with caution in use of certain analgesics, and potential OTC drug-POM-drug interactions (Porteous et al 2005).

The GP should also bear in mind, and be open to hidden pointers, the small number of cases where the patient has knowingly or unknowingly become dependent on an OTC drug, and needs help and ongoing support, ideally in collaboration with the local pharmacists, to address this.

Finally, a recommendation to purchase an OTC medicine, rather than write an NHS prescription would also be a cost-effective way of managing a current presentation as well as educating patients for the future. This is particularly the case for the symptomatic treatment of viral conditions rather than the prescription of an antibiotic. A study has shown that once patients experience resolution of their symptoms without the need for antibiotics they are less likely to consult on subsequent similar occasions (Little et al 1997). The reverse is also true. Awareness of this less immediately obvious outcome may address some GPs' concerns about 'sending patients away'. The use of educational leaflets in lieu of a prescription may also fulfil the need 'to give the patient something'.

The examples above clearly indicate that GP practice should change from the current situation where OTC products are rarely mentioned (Urquhart et al 2004). However, in recommending the purchase of OTC treatment, GPs must bear in mind that, as noted earlier, the OTC licence is often different from the POM licence; this means that both indications and dose may differ. A classic example of this is hydrocortisone one per cent cream which when purchased OTC cannot be used on the face. There are many anecdotes of community pharmacists refusing to sell the product to the customer once they became aware of its ultimate use, to the irritation and inconvenience of all concerned. Research has shown that many GPs are not fully aware of the restrictions on the uses of OTC hydrocortisone (Rogers et al 2004). Education about OTC medicines for health professionals might reduce the potential for patients to receive conflicting information.

## 4.3 Nurses

With changes in management of patients in primary care and the increasing role of nurses in the first line of management of minor illness, the same issues that apply to GPs also apply to nurses as they undertake their consultations. Awareness of OTC medicines and their place in the cost-effective delivery of healthcare should become an important part of their training. This would help ensure that maximum benefit is achieved from OTC medicine use for both the individual patient and the population at large.

The original formulary for independent nurse prescribing was largely based around P and GSL products (in contrast to the extended nurse prescribers' formulary), and it is important that after a first prescription, nurses make it clear to patients that they can access further supplies by direct purchase, if this is financially an option. This demedicalises the care of minor ailments, and educates and empowers the patient.

## 4.4 Collaborative care

OTC use has implications for many healthcare professionals. As it becomes more widespread and effective, it needs to become an integrated part of planned 'NHS' care. Guidelines for treatment, such as those already mentioned, should be coherent across the GP/self-care interface and consistency of information giving to the public is of paramount importance. Educational campaigns directed at the public should be used to promote self-care, and empower the pharmacist as a core member of the NHS team.

For collaborative care to be a reality, shared clinical records, including OTC medicine use need to be considered. This will support team working and allow a comprehensive audit trail of patient management to be maintained. There is some evidence that to record all OTC sales would be burdensome for pharmacies, unwelcome to patients and of concern to GPs because of the perceived increased liability it could bring (Porteous et al 2003). However, as the range of OTC medication continues to grow it may become increasingly important to record OTC use. As such, ways to facilitate recording and share records while acknowledging the perceived barriers should be identified.

# 5. Information and communication

## 5.1 Pharmacoepidemiology of OTC medication use

One of the disadvantages of the lack of a current mechanism to record OTC supply, and by implication use, means that any studies of the pharmacoepidemiology of OTC drugs have to be the subject of dedicated data collection exercises. While these have been shown to be feasible (Sinclair et al 2005; 2002; 2001) they have many limitations including incomplete datasets, short-term data, inability to link to other databases, biases of self-reported data. Thus, there is a lost opportunity for monitoring the ongoing safety of OTC products, newly deregulated products and their use in new populations. This situation is likely to be of increasing concern as products are further deregulated to GSL status and can be supplied from any retail outlet. Advanced IT-based solutions linking purchases to people at point of sale would also not solve the problems, as purchasers are often not the end user.

At the current time, systems of pharmacovigilance include spontaneous reporting via the Yellow Card System and signal generation in various databases followed by event monitoring (Mann 1998) and post marketing surveillance studies. Hypothesis-based case-control and cohort studies (Strom 1989) may also be used.

All of these apply equally to OTC drugs: doctors, pharmacists and nurses can make reports using the Yellow Card System and it is through this that some of the problems with herbal products mentioned earlier have been identified. Likewise cohort studies have already been conducted, as described.

One of the problems with the spontaneous reporting systems is that patients or professionals have to make the link between the drug and the observed (unwanted) effect, and because of the perceived safety of OTC drugs (Porteous 2004) this link is less likely to be made than for prescribed medicines – and it is well recognised that even these events are grossly under reported. Patient reporting of ADRs is being piloted by the MRHA and this might overcome under-identification of events to some extent. It has been argued that patient reporting exposes the system to the potentially crude and incomplete reporting of patients compared to professionals (Egbats et al 1996). Countries, however, in which patient reporting has been introduced have not found this to be the case.

## 5.2 Information for the public

Doctors' and patients' roles in the decision-making process have evolved over recent years to the point where patients will be increasingly encouraged to take more responsibility for their healthcare. There is discussion regarding this issue on the Resourceful Patient website[6]. The site also highlights the amount of information now available, as well as ways of better informing patients with regards to OTC medication.

In order for the public to self-medicate well, to report perceived adverse events, and to answer

---

[6] www.resourcefulpatient.org

questions on drug usage accurately, it is important that they recognise that OTC medicines can be as potent and potentially dangerous as any other drug. Much more information needs to be disseminated to the public about this. The environment in which OTC drugs can be sold, in particular those available from general sales outlets, and the trust the public has in the UK's regulatory system, has resulted in a sense of complacency about the safety of OTC drugs. This leads to a general lack of respect for the medicine, an unwillingness to accept advice or supply controls, a failure to recognise an OTC medicine as a medicine, or to consider it as a cause of unexplained symptoms.

Ways of communicating information to the public include the NHS Direct guide, now included in the Thomson Local Directory and delivered to all households in England, websites such as www.medicinechestonline.com, and of course advice from professionals. The Medicines Partnership Initiative (see www.medicines-partnership.org) has also been instrumental in building relationships between the public and healthcare professionals, including initiatives such as the annual Ask About Medicines Week. In order for the public to be ready to provide the necessary information to pharmacy staff, so that they can support appropriate safe and effective OTC medicine use, they must understand the justification for this apparent breach of their privacy and self-determination. Likewise, they will need to accept the transfer of information about their OTC use to their clinical records. Health Promotion Departments and networks such as the NHS Public Health Practitioners and of course the community pharmacy network can also be used to inform the public. IT based options might include national and local government websites such as NHS Health Scotland, or equivalents in England and Wales.

Finally, it must be remembered that individuals will have differing information needs depending on both their demographics (for example age, gender and educational level) and the health item in question. These differing needs must be identified and met. The Resourceful Patient website is a good source for a discussion of these issues.

## 5.3 Records of OTC purchases
Some pharmacists keep records of OTC purchases on their computerised patient medication records. Research on this is sparse but suggests that a minority of pharmacists do so. The new community pharmacy contractual framework for England introduced a limited record keeping requirement for OTC medicines within 'essential services' from April 2005. Pharmacists are asked to make a record of OTC sales where the patient is known to the pharmacy (the implication being that of a 'regular' customer) and the pharmacist considers it clinically relevant to do so (Pharmaceutical Services Negotiating Committee 2004). There has been no public discussion to date on the practical implementation of such record keeping but there is an opportunity to involve other health professionals and the public in doing so over the coming months. If the trend for POM to P switches of medicines to treat long-term conditions continues, such pharmacy records could become the sole clinical record of their use. Patient safety would be maximised by the joining up of pharmacy systems to the NHS electronic patient record spine.

## 5.4 Shared patient records

NHS programmes for IT propose a single electronic patient record. Inclusion of OTC medicines as an essential piece of information on this record could be a convenient and practical way to overcome some of the disadvantages for OTC medicines articulated in this report. In England NHS Direct Online is piloting My HealthSpace, a patient accessible electronic record. Patients will be able to look at their personal health record and there will be an area where the patient can enter their own information (www.healthspace.nhs.uk). The potential use of My HealthSpace for regular and long-term OTC use could be explored.

Sharing information between professional groups would also support selection and use of appropriate OTC medicine. For example, access to medical records by the pharmacist would aid appropriate 'OTC' diagnosis and reduce the possibility of contra-indicated use, therapeutic duplication, or drug interactions between prescribed and purchased medicines. For the traditional prescriber it should likewise reduce therapeutic duplication, or drug interactions between prescribed and purchased medicines, as well as contributing to a holistic patient history, prompting an understanding of unexpected new symptoms. Sharing information between pharmacists and between pharmacists and other prescribers would also prevent overuse and misuse as patients would no longer be able to go from one pharmacy to another purchasing repeat supplies of medicines.

If this approach were to be implemented, consensus would be required on exactly what information was to be shared and with whom. While pharmacists would welcome access to the whole record, patients and GPs would prefer only subsets of information to be shared, for example the medication record, or main diagnoses only. These articulated concerns are not a reason for delaying this development, but they highlight the need for early education of all stakeholders on the benefits to be gained (Porteous et al 2003). Recognising that IT developments are complex, and often delayed for a range of technical, political and financial reasons, a patient held record might be an interim option. Patient held records have been successfully used previously for shared care arrangements between general practice and secondary care, for example, in antenatal care, or diabetes. Although the most widely used have been paper based, optically readable cards, and microchip systems have also been piloted, and may well be more convenient and acceptable. These could be adapted to include a subset of relevant information focusing on diagnoses and medication history only, but specifically including OTC use. As well as supporting safe and effective use of OTC medicines integrated with NHS care, it should also educate patients as to the potency of OTC medicines, and their equal status with other medicines.

# 6. Conclusions

Self-management of acute, intermittent and long-term conditions is likely to become more extensive in the future. Long-term self-treatment to prevent ill health will also become more prevalent. Obtaining benefit while managing potential risks will continue to be key issues. With greater self-treatment of long-term conditions more effective ways will need to be found to manage the interface between individuals' NHS care and their self-care. A balance needs to be struck between safety and patient autonomy. Greater patient and public involvement in formulating both policy and practice will be needed. Education programmes for the public and for health professionals will be necessary.

# 7. Recommendations

## Integrating self-care with the NHS

- A more strategic approach to POM to P switches could enable priorities relating to patient need to be identified and implemented, particularly in relation to long-term conditions.

- Work on POM to P switches needs to be integrated with the current NHS activity to develop and support self-care, particularly the work programme on management of long-term conditions.

- As more potent medicines switch from P to GSL further research is needed to enable pharmacovigilance, assess the effects of the lack of associated professional input and difficulties in achieving record linkage and patient tracing.

- A readily accessible source bringing together the evidence on OTC medicines could provide decision support for patients and healthcare providers. Such a source should address both benefits and risks of OTC treatment, and be internet or paper based.

## Healthcare professionals

- Healthcare providers, particularly those who are prescribing, need to know about available OTC medicines and their licensed indications and doses. Education programmes during basic training and as part of CPD are needed. Multidisciplinary approaches would also increase mutual inter-professional understanding.

- It is important that prescribers routinely ask patients about OTC medicines they are using. Computer based decision support could facilitate this.

## The public

- Consideration could be given to educational courses on self-management of common illnesses for children and adults.

- Education about self-care could support parents from the birth of their first child, to develop knowledge and confidence about when to seek advice.

- As OTC medicines evolve there is a need for education about their changing nature and role. A general leaflet, available from pharmacies, could describe trends in OTC availability, point out advantages and drawbacks, and encourage patient reporting of suspected ADRs.

- Patient information leaflets and package information for any new OTC medicine should involve users in their development.

- Formal user testing of both patient information leaflets and package labelling should be a requirement for any medicine switched from POM to P or from P to GSL.

- Facilitating patient reporting of suspected adverse reactions to OTC medicines as part of self-management could improve surveillance. A reporting form should be included in medicines switched from POM to P or from P to GSL.

## Record keeping

- Heathcare providers and medicine users need to discuss the extent to which formal record keeping for OTC medicines should be implemented. There is a balance to be struck between autonomy and safety.

- Including OTC treatment in the NHS core electronic patient record could make an important contribution to improving patient safety.

- The development of 'My HealthSpace' for patients to record their health information also offers promise in relation to OTC treatment.

- In the meantime, a hard copy patient held record offers a means for patients to share information about OTC treatments with healthcare providers.

# Glossary

| | |
|---|---|
| CPD | Continuing Professional Development |
| FDA | Food and Drug Administration (USA) |
| GSL | General Sales List medicine |
| MAS | Minor Ailment Scheme |
| MCA | Medicine Counter Assistant |
| MHRA | Medicines and Healthcare products Regulatory Authority (UK) |
| NeLH | National electronic Library for Health |
| NICE | National Institute for Clinical Effectiveness |
| NPfIT | National Programme for IT (Now 'Connecting for Health') |
| OTC | Over-the-counter |
| P | Pharmacy only medicine |
| PEFR | Peak Expiratory Flow Rate |
| PGD | Patient Group Direction |
| POM | Prescription only medicine |
| PRODIGY | NHS prescribing guidelines (www.prodigy.nhs.uk) |

# References

Adcock H (2001) OTC medicines misuse and addiction: what can pharmacists do to help? *The Pharmaceutical Journal* **267:** 457.

Adcock H (2004) Self care goes under the microscope. *The Pharmaceutical Journal* **273:** 715.

Anderson MR, Klink K & Cohrssen A (2004) Evaluation of vaginal complaints. *JAMA* **291**: 1368.

Anonymous (1994a) Protocols and staff training to be added to Code of Ethics. *The Pharmaceutical Journal* **252:** 124.

Anonymous (1994b) Introductory protocol points. *The Pharmaceutical Journal* **253:** 805.

Anonymous (1994c) Society issues press release on protocols. *The Pharmaceutical Journal* **251:** 127.

Anonymous (1995) POM-to-P shift proposed for budesonide and P-to-POM for carbaryl. *The Pharmaceutical Journal* **255:** 138.

Anonymous (1997) Terfenadine switches back to POM. *The Pharmaceutical Journal* **259:** 316.

Anonymous (2000) Third pharmacy-based EHC pilot about to start in Derbyshire. *The Pharmaceutical Journal* **264:** 712.

Anonymous (2001) Pharmacy-based head lice management. *The Pharmaceutical Journal* **267:** 317.

Anonymous (2002) Pharmacists in Scotland target low income pregnant women who smoke. *The Pharmaceutical Journal* **269:** 182.

Aronson JK (2004) Over-the-counter medicines. *Br J Clin Pharmacol* **58:** 231-4.

Barnett NL, Denham MJ & Francis SA (2000) Over-the-counter medicines and the elderly. *J R Coll Physicians Lond* **34:** 445-6.

Bayliss E & Rutter P (2004) General practitioners' views on recent and proposed medicine switches from POM to P. *The Pharmaceutical Journal* **273:** 819-21.

Beitz R, Doren M & Knopf H et al (2004) Over-the-counter self medication in Germany. *Bundesgesundheitsblatt Gesundheitsforschung Gesundheitsschutz* **47:** 1043-50.

Birchley N & Conroy S (2002) Parental management of over-the-counter medicines. *Paediatr Nurs* **14:** 24-8.

Bissell P, Ward PR & Noyce P (2001) The dependent consumer: reflections on accounts of the risks of non-prescription medicines. *Health* **5:** 5-30.

Blenkinsopp A & Noyce P (2002) *Minor illness management in primary care: a review of NHS community pharmacy NHS schemes.* Department of Medicines Management: Keele University. www.keele.ac.uk/depts/mm/Publications/documents/MinorIllnessDec2002.pdf (accessed 14/1/05).

Bond CM & Grimshaw JM (1994) Clinical guidelines for the treatment of dyspepsia in community pharmacies. *The Pharmaceutical Journal* **252:** 228-9.

Bousquet J (on behalf of Aria workshop members) (2004) ARIA in the pharmacy; management of allergic rhinitis symptoms in the pharmacy. *Allergy* **59:** 373-87.

Bradley C, Kenkre J & Tobias R et al (1996) GPs' rate of recommending over the counter drugs varies. *BMJ* **313:** 115-6.

Bradley CP, Riaz A & Tobias RS et al (1998) Patient attitudes to over-the-counter drugs and possible professional responses to self-medication. *Fam Pract* **15:** 44-50.

Branstad JO, Kamil I & Lilja J et al (1994) When topical hydrocortisone became an OTC drug in Sweden – a study of the users and their information sources. *Soc Sci Med* **39:** 207-12.

Brass EP (2001) Changing the status of drugs from prescription to over-the-counter availability. *New England Journal of Medicine* **345:** 810-6.

Brass EP (2004) Consumer behaviour in the setting of over-the-counter statin availability. *Am J Cardiol* **94:** 22F-29F.

Breckenridge A (2002) CSM advice on liver toxicity associated with kava-kava and proposed regulatory action by the government committee on safety of medicines. CEM/CMO/2002/10.

British Market Research Bureau (1997) Everyday Health Care. Proprietary Association of Great Britain: London. www.pagb.co.uk/pagb/primarysections/marketinformation/ otcconsumeresearch.htm

Checkland K (2002) The gap between practice and research. bmj.bmjjournals.com/cgi/eletters/324/7333/329

Cohen JP, Paquette C & Cairns CP (2005) Switching prescription drugs to over the counter. *BMJ* **330:** 39-41.

Committee for Safety of Medicines and Medicines Control Agency (1992) Astemizole and terfenadine. *Current problems in pharmacovigilance.* London: Committee on Safety of Medicines.

Committee on Safety of Medicines (2000) Reminder St John's Wort interactions. *Current Problems in Pharmacovigilance.* London: Committee on Safety of Medicines: May 26:5

Committee on Safety of Medicines (2004) Advice on the use of celecoxib and other selective COX-2 inhibitors in the light of concerns about cardiovascular safety. *Letter to health care professionals Celecoxib* epinet 20/12/04.

Davies NM & Jamali F (2004) COX-2 selective inhibitors cardiac toxicity: getting to the heart of the matter. *Journal of Pharmaceutical Science* **7:** 332-6

Department of Health (2004) Making the best use of the pharmacy workforce. (page 14).

Egberts TCG, Smulders M & de Koning FHP et al (1996) Can adverse drug reactions be detected earlier? A comparison of reports by patients and professionals. *BMJ* **313:** 530-1.

Emmerton L & Shaw J (2002) The influence of pharmacy staff in non-prescription medicine sales. *Int J Pharm Pract* **10:** 101-6.

Erwin J, Britten N & Jones R (1996) General practitioners' views on over the counter sales by community pharmacists. *BMJ* **312:** 617-8.

Erwin J, Britten N & Jones R (1997) General practitioners' views on over the counter availability of $H_2$ antagonists. *Br J Gen Pract* **47:** 99-102.

European Community (1992) Directive for medicines classification. 92/26/EEC of 31 March 1992 concerning the classification for the supply of medicinal products for human use, OJ L 113, 30 April 1992.

Fendrick AM, Shaw M & Schnactel B et al (2004) Self-selection and use patterns of over-the-counter omeprazole for frequent heartburn. *Clin Gastroenterol Hepatol* **2:** 17-21.

Fenichel RR (2004) Which drugs should be available over the counter. *BMJ* **329:** 182-3.

Gore P & Madhavan S (1993) Credibility of the sources of information for non-prescription medicines. *J Soc Admin Pharm* **10:** 109-22.

Grieve D (2004) Over Count statistical returns.

Hassell K, Noyce P & Rogers A (1999) A review of factors that influence the use of community pharmacy as a primary health care resource. *Int J Pharm Pract* **7:** 51-9.

Hassell K, Whittington Z & Cantrill J et al (2001) Managing demand: transfer of management of self limiting conditions from general practice to community pharmacies. *BMJ* **323:** 146-7.

Henley E & Wenzel-Wamhoff J. Teaching medical students about over-the-counter medication. Med Educ (2000) **34:** 580-2

Hughes GF, McElnay JC & Hughes CM et al (1999) Abuse/misuse of non-prescription drugs. *Pharm World Sci* **21:** 251-5.

Kilby S (2005) Royal Pharmaceutical Society of Great Britain (Personal communication).

Lefterover A & Getov I (2004) Study on consumers' preferences and habits for over the counter analgesics use. *Cent Eur J Public Health* **12:** 43-5.

Li Wan Po A & Zhang WY (1996) Paracetamol-codeine combinations versus paracetamol alone. *BMJ* **313:** 1209.

Little P, Gould C & Williamson I et al (1997) Reattendance and complications in a randomised trial of prescribing strategies for sore throat: the medicalising effect of prescribing antibiotics *BMJ*. **315:** 350-2.

Mann R & Andrews E Pharmacovigilance handbook. CHIPSBOOKS

Matheson C, Bond CM & Pitcairn J (2002) Misuse of over the counter medicines from community pharmacies: a population survey of Scottish Pharmacies. *The Pharmaceutical Journal* **269:** 66-8.

Matheson C & Bond CM (1995) Lower gastrointestinal symptoms. *The Pharmaceutical Journal* **253:** 656-8.

McBride AJ, Pates R & Ramadan R et al (2003) Delphi survey of experts' opinions on strategies used by community pharmacists to reduce over-the-counter drug misuse. *Addiction* **98:** 487.

Medicines and Healthcare products Regulatory Agency (MHRA). *Policy on legal status of medicines.* www.medicines.mhra.gov.uk/ourwork/licensingmeds/legalstatus/legstat.htm (accessed 14/1/05).

Moore N, Van Ganse E & Le Parc JM et al (1999) The PAIN study: paracetamol, aspirin and ibuprofen new tolerability study. *Clinical Drug Investment* **18:** 89-98.

Morgan, Oliver & Griffiths et al (2005) Impact of paracetamol pack size restrictions on poisoning from paracetamol in England and Wales: an observational study. *J Public Health Med* **27:** 19-24.

Morley A, Jepson MH & Edwards C et al (1984) Should pharmacists treat minor ailments? *Chemist and Druggist.* 82-4.

Morris CJ, Cantrill JA & Weiss MC (1997) One simple question should be enough: consumers' perceptions of pharmacy protocols. *Int J Pharm Pract* **5:** 64-71.

National Pharmaceutical Association (2004) Implementing a Minor Ailment scheme: a practical toolkit for primary care organisations.

Pates R, McBride A & Li S et al (2002) Misuse of over the counter medicines: a survey of community pharmacies in a South Wales health authority. *The Pharmaceutical Journal* **268:** 179-82.

Payne K, Ryan-Woolley B & Noyce P (1998) Role of consumer attributes in predicting the uptake of medicines deregulation and National Health Service prescribing in the United Kingdom. *Int J Pharm Pract* **6:** 150-8.

Phelan M, Akram G & Lewis M et al (2002) A community pharmacy based survey of users of over-the-counter sleep aids. *The Pharmaceutical Journal* **269:** 287-90.

Pillitteri JL, Kozlowski LT & Person DC et al (1994) Over-the-counter sleep aids: widely used but rarely studied. *J Subst Abuse* **6:** 315-23.

Porteous T, Bond CM & Hannaford P et al (2005) How and why are non-prescription analgesics used in Scotland? *Family Practice.*

Porteous T, Bond CM & Sinclair H et al (2002) *Non-prescribed analgesics: how and why are they used?* Report to Chief Scientist Office. London: HMSO.

Porteous T, Bond CM & Hannaford P et al (2003) Electronic transfer of prescription related information: comparing the views of patients, GPs and pharmacists. *Br J Gen Pract* **53:** 204-9.

Porteous T, Bond CM & Duthie I et al (1997) Guidelines for the treatment of hayfever and other allergic conditions of the upper respiratory tract. *The Pharmaceutical Journal* **259:** 62-5.

Porteous T, Bond CM & Duthie I et al (1998) Guidelines for the treatment of self limiting upper respiratory tract ailments. *The Pharmaceutical Journal* **260:** 134-9.

Pradel FG, Hartzema AG & Mutran EJ et al (1999) Physician over-the-counter prescribing patterns: an analysis of the National Ambulatory Medical Care Survey. *Ann Pharmacother* **33:** 400-5.

Prayle D & Brazier M (1998) Supply of medicines: paternalism, autonomy and reality. *J Med Ethics* **24:** 93-8

Proprietary Association of Great Britain (2004). *Self Care Review.* London: PAGB.

Protocols and staff training to be added to Code of Ethics. *The Pharmaceutical Journal* **252:** 124.

Rallapalli KC & Smith MC (1994) OTC drug advertising-information content. *J Soc Admin Pharm* **11:** 139-47.

Rogers PJ, Wood SM & Garrett E et al (2004) Awareness and recommendation of over-the-counter topical steroids by general practitioners and community pharmacists. *Int J Pharm Pract* **12:** R14.

Roumie CL & Griffin MR (2004) Over the counter analgesics in older adults: a call for improved labelling and consumer education. *Drugs Aging* **21:** 485-98.

Royal Pharmaceutical Society of Great Britain (2000) Prescription only medicines reclassified to pharmacy only medicines.

Royal Pharmaceutical Society of Great Britain (2004) *Code of Ethics Service Specification.* 10 July 2004 no 98.

Royal Pharmaceutical Society of Great Britain. *Potential candidates for reclassification from POM to P.* www.rpsgb.org.uk/members/pdfs/pomtopreclasslist.pdf#xml=http://fm315.facility.pipex.com/cgi-bin/pdf_hl?STEMMER=en&RGB=ff00ff&WORDS=pom+p+&DB=RPSGB-members&URL=http://www.rpsgb.org.uk/members/pdfs/pomtopreclasslist.pdf (accessed 14/1/05).

Royal Pharmaceutical Society of Great Britain. *Reclassification strategy.* www.rpsgb.org.uk/members/pdfs/pomtopreclassinftr.pdf#xml=http://fm315.facility.pipex.com/cgi-bin/pdf_hl?STEMMER=en&RGB=ff00ff&WORDS=pom+p+&DB=RPSGB-members&URL=http://www.rpsgb.org.uk/members/pdfs/pomtopreclassinftr.pdf (accessed 14/1/05).

Sansgiry S, Sharp WT & Sansgiry SS (1999) Department of Pharmacy Practice and Administrative Sciences, College of Pharmacy, Idaho State University. *Health Mark Q* **17:** 7-18.

Sansgiry SS & Cady PS (1996) How the elderly and young adults differ in the decision-making process of non-prescription medication purchases. *Health Mark Q* **14:** 3-21.

Schafheutle E, Cantrill, J & Nicolson M et al (1996) Insights into the choice between self medication and a doctor's prescription: a study of hay fever sufferers. *Int J Pharm Pract* **4:** 156-61.

Schafheutle EI, Noyce PR & Sheehy C et al (2002) Users and costs of the Scottish Direct Supply of Medicines scheme. *Int J Pharm Pract* **10:** R63.

Shaw J & Baker M (2004) Expert patient – dream or nightmare? *BMJ* **328:** 723-4

Shih YC, Prasad M & Luce BR (2002) The effect on social welfare of a switch of second-generation antihistamines from prescription to over-the-counter status: a microeconomic analysis. *Clinical Therapy* **24:** 701-16.

Sihvo S, Hemminki E & Ahonen R (1999) Physicians' attitudes toward reclassifying drugs as over-the-counter. *Med Care* **37:** 518-25.

Sinclair H, (2003) (personal communication) from Sinclair H, Urquhart G & Hannaford P. The use of non-prescription medicines by GP attendees. Forthcoming publication based on BMed Sci thesis, University of Aberdeen (GU) 2001.

Sinclair H, Lawton S & Bond CM et al. Patient reported satisfaction of treatments for allergic rhinitis provided from community pharmacies. [Submitted to IJPP]

Sinclair HK, Bond CM & Hannaford PC (2000) Over the counter ibuprofen: how and why is it used? *Int J Pharm Pract* **8:** 121-7.

Sinclair HK, Bond CM & Hannaford PC (2001) Long term follow up studies of users of non-prescription medicines purchased from community pharmacies: some methodological issues. *Drug Safety* **24:** 929-39.

Sleath B, Rubin RH & Campbell W et al (2001) Physician-patient communication about over-the-counter medications. *Soc Sci Med* **53:** 357-69.

Spencer JA & Edwards C (1992) Pharmacy beyond the dispensary: general practitioners' views. *BMJ* **304:** 1670-2.

Stevenson FA, Britten N & Barry CA et al (2003) Self-treatment and its discussion in medical consultations: how is medical pluralism managed in practice? *Soc Sci Med* **57:** 513-27.

Strom BL (1989) Choosing among the available approaches for pharmacoepidemiologic studies. In: B L Strom (ed.) *Pharmacoepidemiology.* New York: Churchill Livingstone: pp 245-56.

Taylor J (1994) Reasons consumers do not ask for advice on non-prescription medicines. *Int J Pharm Pract* **2:** 209-14

Urquhart G, Sinclair HK & Hannaford PC (2004) The use of non-prescription medicines by general practitioner attendees. *Pharmacoepidemiology and Drug Safety* **13:** 773-9.

Walker A, Watson MC & Grimshaw J et al (2004) Applying the theory of planned behaviour to pharmacists' beliefs and intentions about the treatment of vaginal candidiasis with non prescription medicines. *Family Practice* **21:** 1-7.

Walker R, Evans S & Kirkland D (2003) Evaluation of 'Care at the pharmacy' in Gwent on the management of self limiting conditions and workload of a general medical practice. *Int J Pharm Pract* **11:** R7.

Watson MC, Grimshaw JM & Bond CM et al (2002) Oral versus intra-vaginal imidazole and triazole anti-fungal agents for the treatment of uncomplicated vulvovaginal candidiasis (thrush): a systematic review. *BJOG* **109:** 85-95.

Watson MC, Grimshaw JM & Bond CM et al (2002) Oral versus intra-vaginal imidazole and triazole anti-fungal treatment of uncomplicated vulvovaginal candidiasis (thrush). *Cochrane Database Syst Rev* **4:** CD002845 (latest version 28 May 2001).

Watson MC, Bond CM & Grimshaw JM et al (2002) Educational strategies to promote evidence-based community pharmacy practice: a cluster randomised controlled trial (RCT). *Family Practice* **19:** 529-36.

Watson MC & Bond CM on behalf of the members of the Grampian Evidence Based Community Pharmacy Guidelines Group (2003). Evidence-based guidelines for the over-the-counter treatment of vulvovaginal candidiasis. *Pharmacy World and Science* **25:** 129-34.

Watson MC & Bond CM (2004) The evidence based supply of non-prescription medicines: barriers and beliefs. *Int J Pharm Pract* **12:** 65-72.

Whittington Z, Cantrill J & Hassell KJ et al (2001) Community pharmacy management of minor conditions – the 'care at the Chemist' scheme. *The Pharmaceutical Journal* **266:** 425-8.

Wiesenfeld HC, Lowry DLB & Phillips Heine R et al (2001) Self collection of vaginal swabs for the detection of chlamydia, gonorrhea and trichomoniasis. *Sexually Transmitted Diseases* **28:** 321-25.

# Further resources

**Relevant websites – for the public, for professionals**

Support for self care: www.dh.gov.uk/selfcare

Evidence based treatment – versions for patients and health professionals: BestTreatments (access via www.nhsdirect.nhs.uk)

Evidence-based guidelines: PRODIGY (www.prodigy.nhs.uk); SIGN (www.sign.ac.uk)

Manufacturers' directory of OTC products (including dietary supplements): www.medicinechestonline.com

Medicines Guides – new leaflets produced by multi-stakeholder group. Under development www.medguides.medicines.org.uk

The Resourceful Patient website: www.resourcefulpatient.org